G000060148

915 00000289018

Flo's Fro and Curls

A Book on Growing and Nurturing Your Baby's Hair From Birth

Written By: April Laugh

Edit By: Adeboro Odunlami

Flo's Fro and Curls By April Laugh

Written By: April Laugh
Edit By: Adeboro Odunlami

www.growingwithflo.co.uk
Email: hello@growingwithflo.co.uk

Today is wash day!
One of my bestest bestest days.

Mama takes my hair out of its rows and it
makes a big afro

Wow, wizzily wow!
What beautiful hair I've got

I love my hair and all my curls

The way it bounces and sometimes twirls

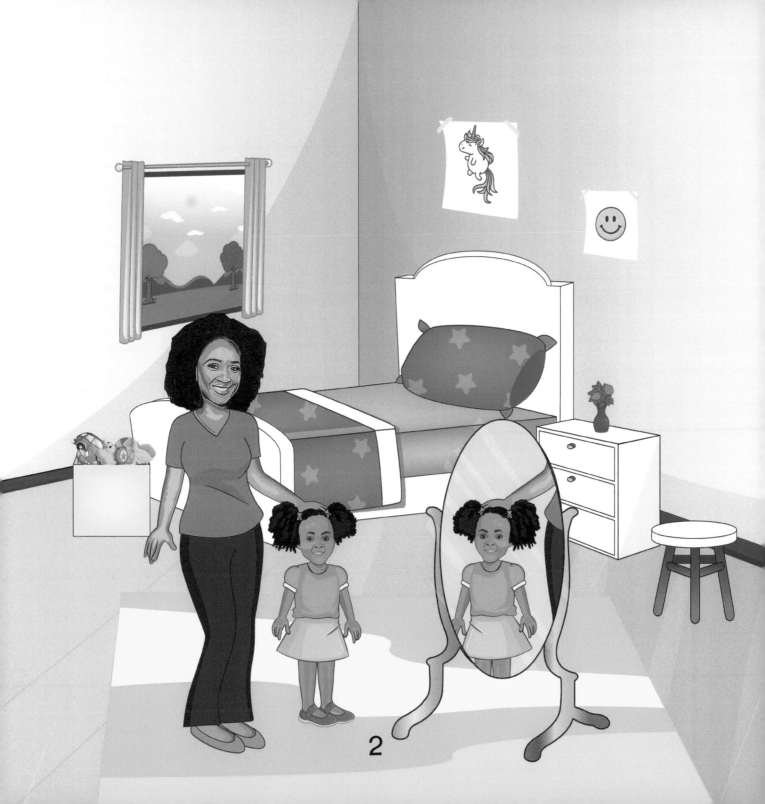

Now, mama says

"Sit. Put up your tiny feet."
"Get ready for the wash day drive.
Remember to count one to five. "

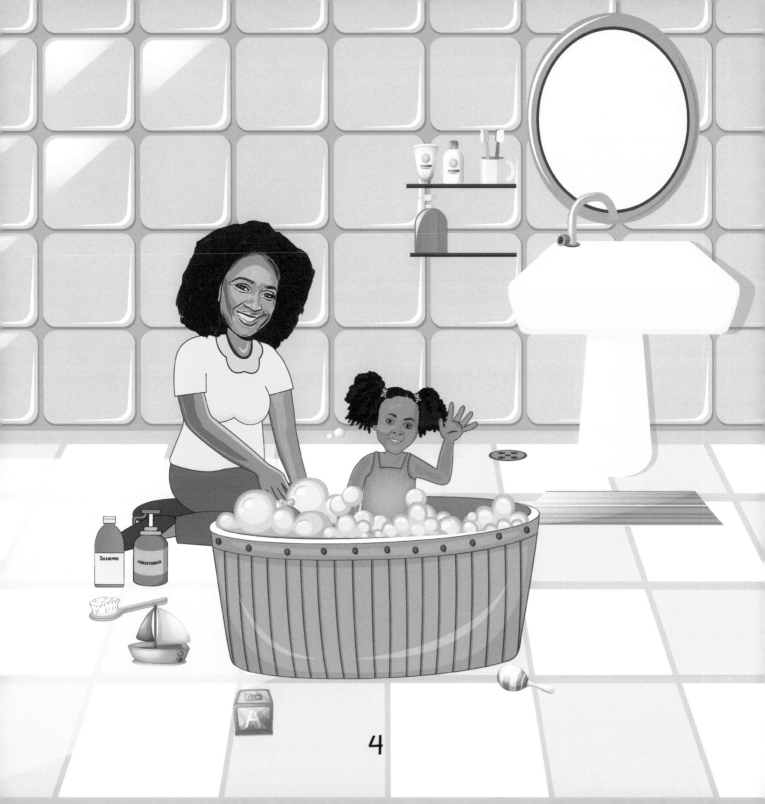

1.

I gather all my products

My shampoo & conditioner to wash washy wash

My oil & moisturiser, make my hair soft soft soft

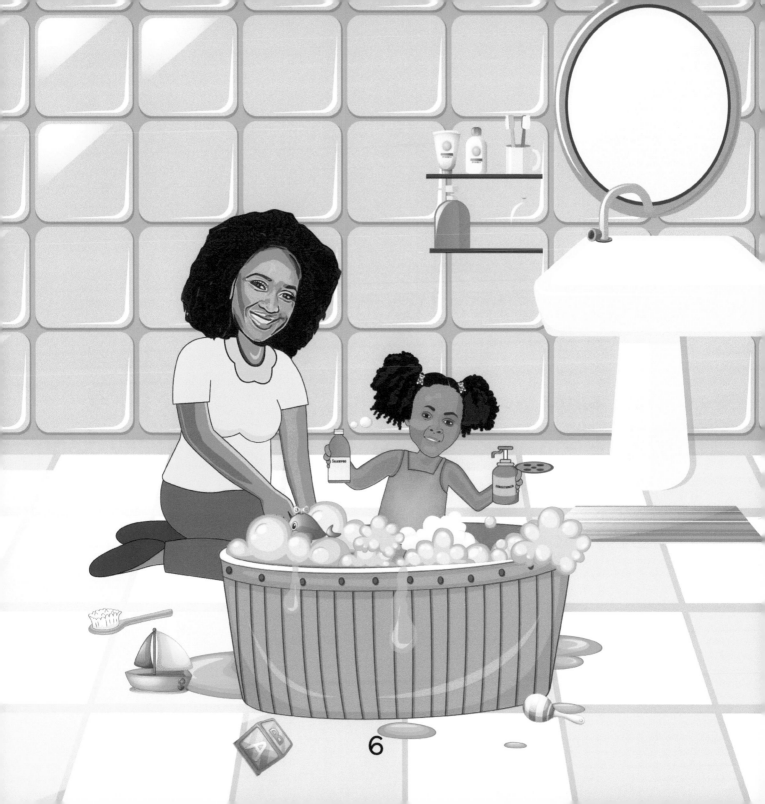

2.

Now, I wash my hair

First some water – ouuu my scalp feels so good
Then some shampoo – ahhh my hair feels squeaky clean
Then some conditioner – ouuuu it softens up my hair
Last, more water – ahhh this feels soo good.

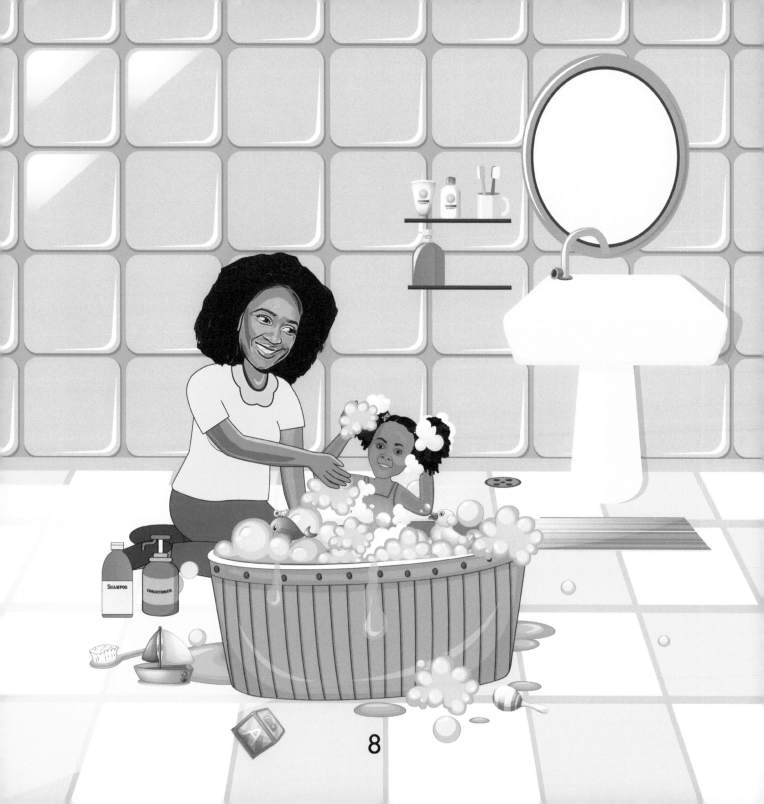

3.

Now, I dry my hair

But just a teeny weeny bit
My hair goes from drip drippy drip
To a gentle damp damp damp

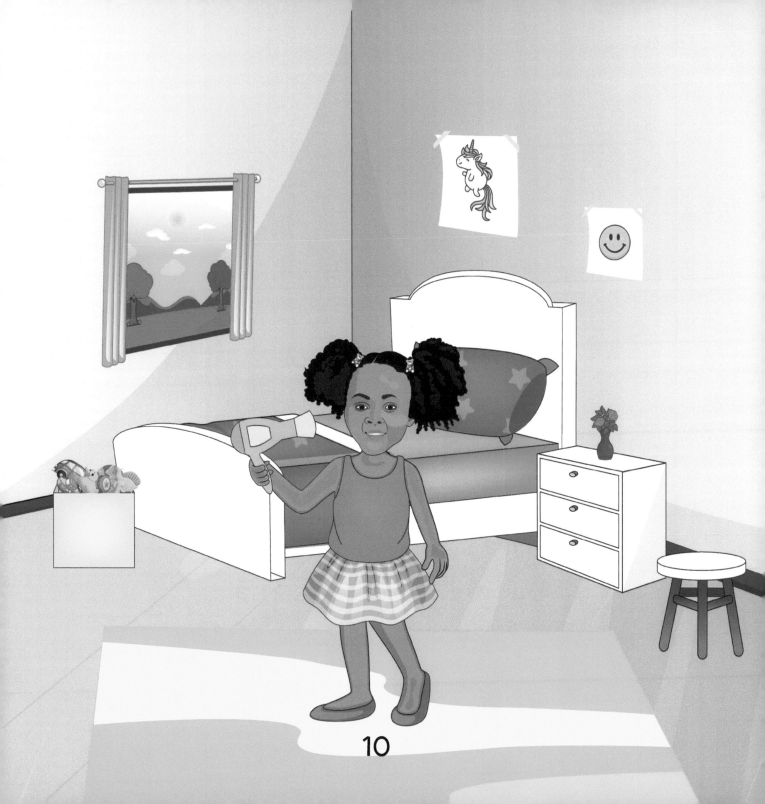

10

4.

Now I moisturize

Squish in the oil
Splat in the moisturizer
Into the roots and all the sides
Some time it may take
Some strength it may take
But well-moisturized hair
Will not break

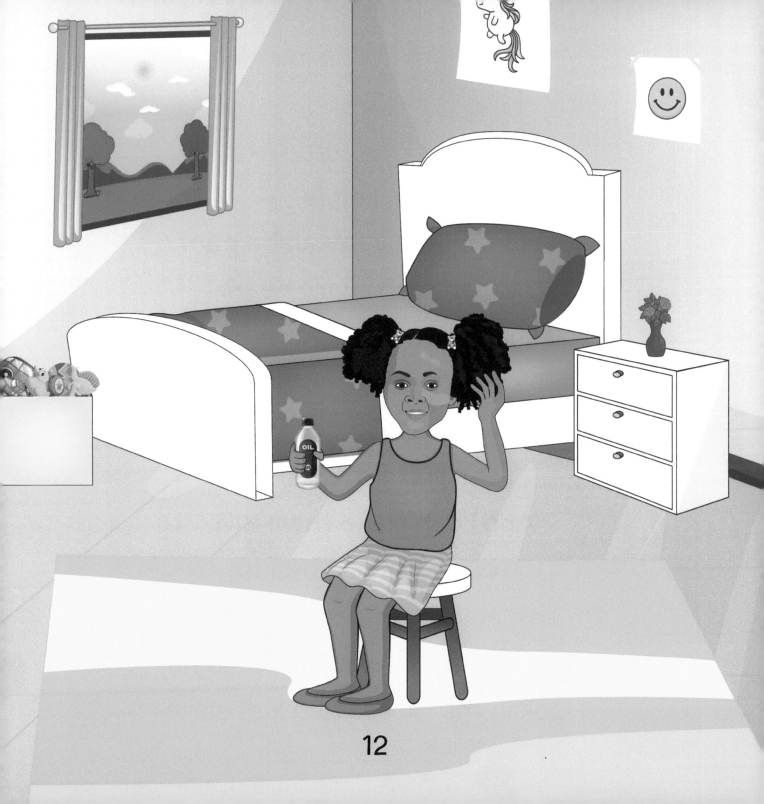

5.

Now, I style

Here comes my favourite part

I love it with all my heart

Do you know what I can do with my hair?

I can make cornrows

I can make twists

I can make them small

And I can make them BIG

I can put some beads

Or just leave my hair out as I please

When I make my protective style

I look in the mirror and just smile

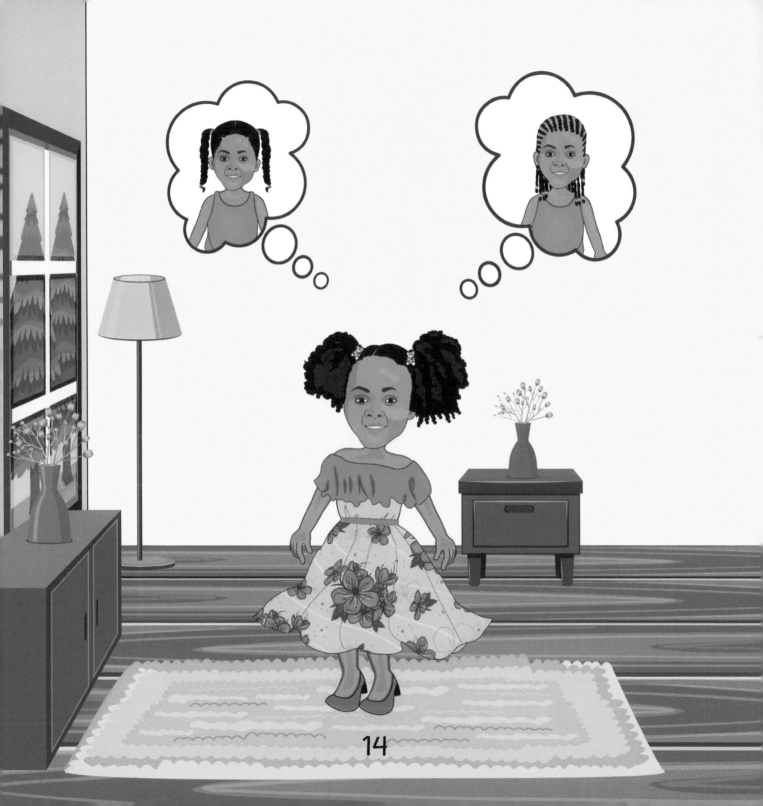

14

Now that wash day is over
I give mama a little kiss
To tell her I love her

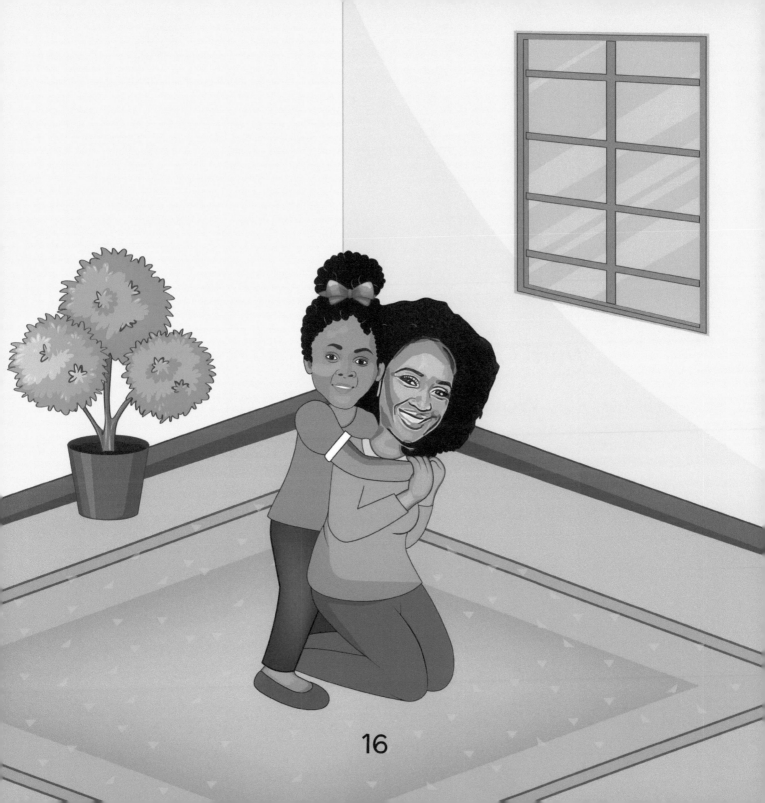

Wait! One more look in the mirror

Wow. I see a beautiful girl

and her beautiful hair.

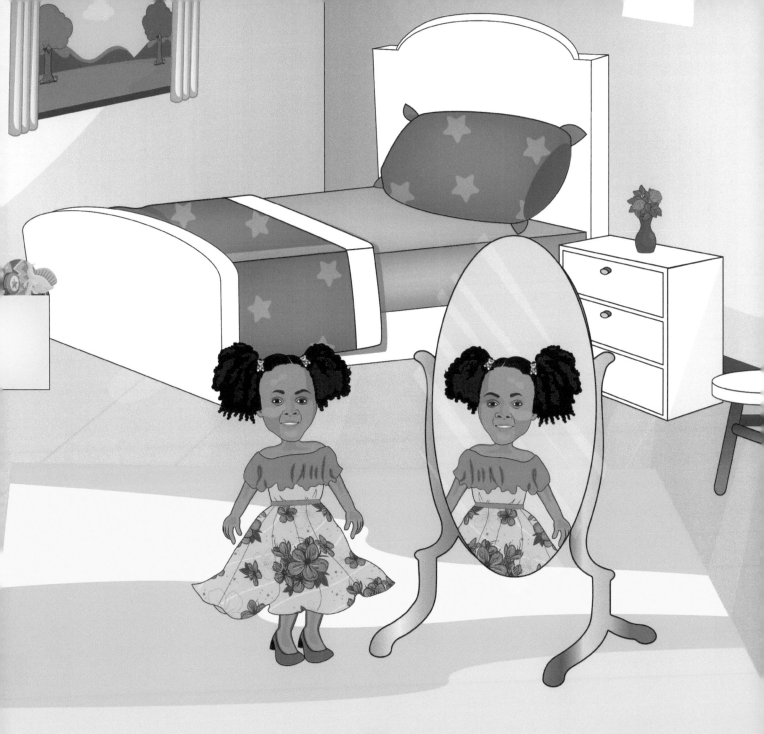

THE END

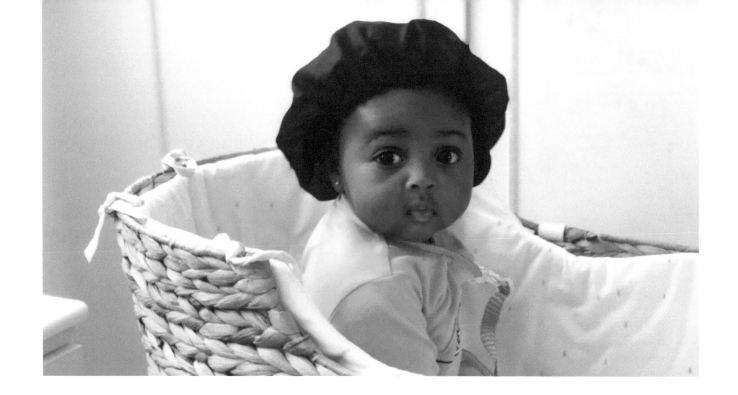

Note To Parents
Hello Mama (& Papa)

I truly understand what it means to desire to be a present and intentional parent; to give the best to your children whilst balancing all your other responsibilities. As you may know, I have two toddlers, two businesses and a host of other responsibilities. Yet our kids deserve care and so do their hair. Below, I have written a short note to help you understand a couple of things about your baby's hair as you follow the prompts in the book.

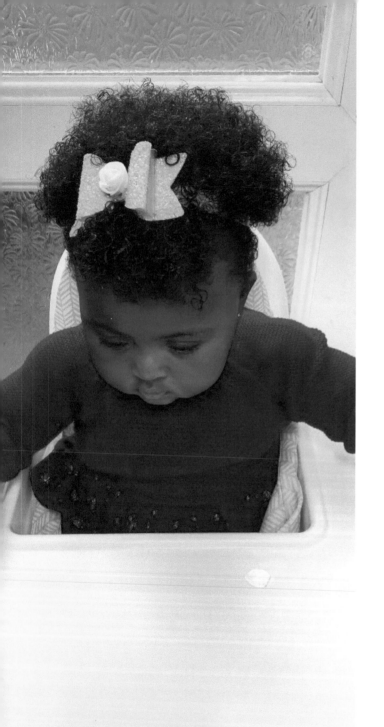

I wish you all the very best in your hair care journey!

What To Know About Your Baby's Hair

Chances are that if you're holding this book, you are African, or of African descent or at least have an African child in your care. So, you already know that African hair is different and peculiar and not all routines or products on the internet work for our hair.

This book contributes to the growing wealth of research on African hair. **The first thing I want you to note about your baby's hair is that it's no**

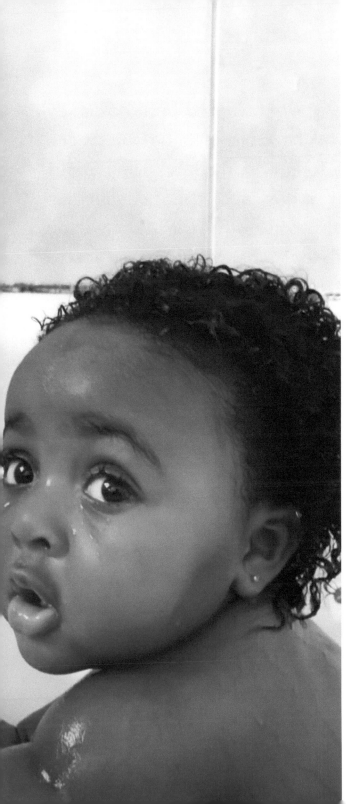

other person's hair but your baby's.
I've come to find that even when generic routines and products are prescribed for hair care, one still had to understand the particular hair mass and know what it likes. I know some people who swear by a product like Coconut Oil and some other people who have to avoid it like a plague. So know your baby's hair. As you follow the routine illustrated in this book, watch how the hair responds to the different steps or products. Does your baby's hair want you to wash more often or less? Does your baby's hair love warm or lukewarm water?

The second thing I want you to note about your baby's hair is its type. African hair is classified into different types and understanding

22

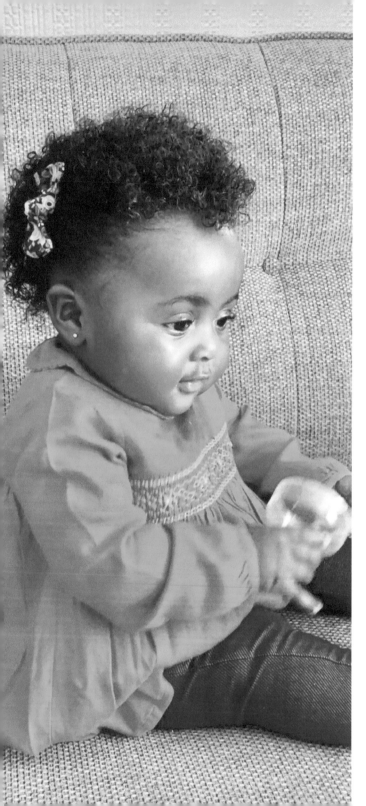

the type of hair your baby has is key to taking care of it better. There are tons of materials online about hair types and the peculiarities that come with caring for the different types, so I'll advise you to check them out. However, if your baby is still below 12 months, it's possible that the hairs on their heads are still 'baby hairs' and the type of your baby's hair has not been fully assumed. That said, this book provides a general routine that can typically be used for baby hair. It's a great template to use until (and most likely, even after), your baby's hair fully assumes its type. In fact, the routine in this book will help your baby's hair develop even better and will help to avoid a streak of unhealthy hair problems as they grow.

The third thing I want you to note about your baby's hair is that it needs love and acceptance. I implore you to not compare your baby's hair to other babies'. Instead, love and accept their hair and teach them to do the same. Remember that their hair is not what defines them or gives them their worth or even their beauty. Whether shaven or full, we are way more than meets the eye. And that's a better confident booster than a luscious mane of hair.

This fourth note is for parents with newborn babies. Newborn hair and skin are soft, sensitive and tender. Hence, special care should be taken when caring for a neonate. Here's a summary of the basic things to do:

- ø Do not wash a newborn's hair daily or use shampoo until they are about 3 months old.
- ø You may use conditioner once in 2 weeks instead.
- ø Please do not style a newborn's hair in tight hairstyles. Nothing that strains their scalps. At least until 6 months.
- ø Use satin pillowcases in bed, car seat, buggy and wherever they nap.

Finally, just a quick guide to routines:

Twice every week:
- ø Co-wash (that is, wash only with a conditioner)
- ø Moisturise

Every two weeks:
- ø Wash with shampoo & conditioner
- ø Moisturise

Every morning & evening:
- ø Moisturise (Water, Hair Oil, Moisturiser)

Every night:
- ø Use a satin pillow/pillow with a satin pillowcase

Please note:
- ø Don't style with any hair accessories that will pull your baby's scalp.
- ø Use attachments and extensions scarcely. Avoid totally if you can.

OKAY, ONE FINAL THING!

The hair, just like many other parts of the body, is just a reflection of a person's health. If your child is healthy, chances are that their hair will be its healthiest version. One way to ensure that your child's hair, skin, immune system, and organs, all function optimally is by healthy eating. It's fruitless to purchase oils, creams and serums that promise hair growth if you don't first tackle the root cause of unhealthy hair. Diet. Routines are great (I stick to the routines in this book religiously), but diet is greater. Good diet + Good routine = Healthy Hair. It would be unfair for me to share Flo's hair routine and not her diet routine.

I have published two very detailed, very rich, very easy-to-follow books titled, 'WhatFloEats', on Flo's diet routine right from 6 months till her current toddler years.

You may shop them here: https://www.growingwithflo.co.uk/shop/

All the best!
Love,

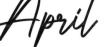

26

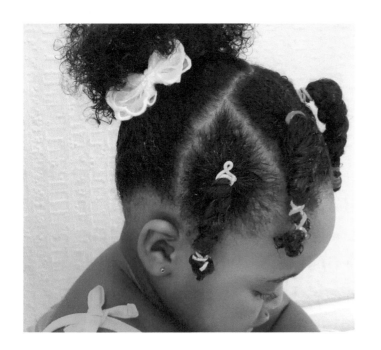

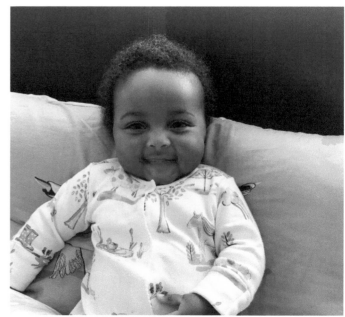

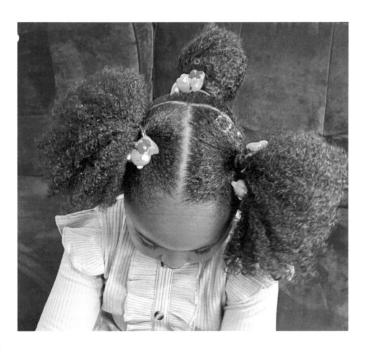

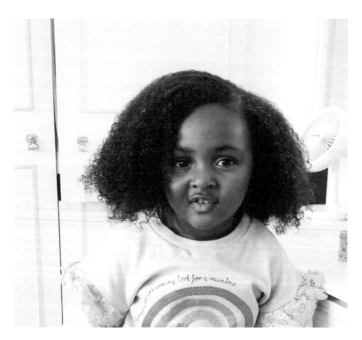

27

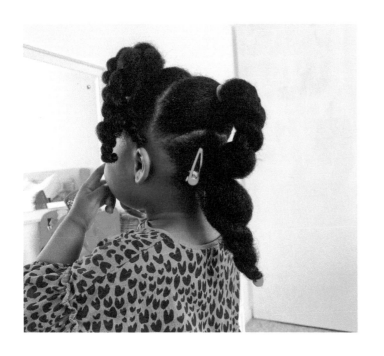
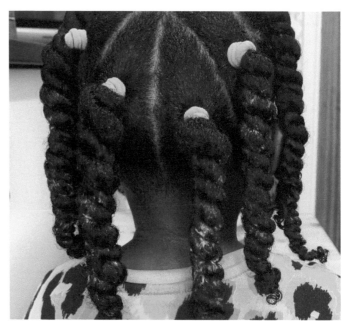
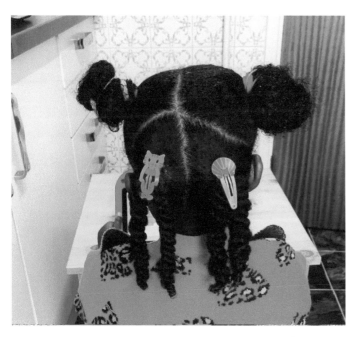
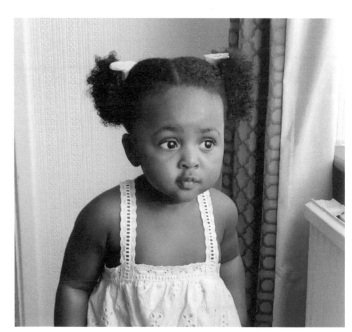

28

Lightning Source UK Ltd.
Milton Keynes UK
UKHW051248180123
415535UK00004B/40